# Suzie Q Gets a BMT

## (Bone Marrow Transplant)

by Dr Sue Futeral-Myrowitz

Illustrations by Penny Myrowitz, age 9 (Dr. Sue's granddaughter)

To order additional copies of this book, contact:
Xlibris
844-714-8691
www.Xlibris.com
Orders@Xlibris.com

ISBN:   Softcover        978-1-6698-0224-2
        EBook            978-1-6698-0253-2

Print information available on the last page

Rev. date: 12/06/2021

This book is dedicated to my family, husband Capp, kids; Jason, Deb, Justin, Rebecca, Mindy Simcha; and grand kids: Penny, Shane, Reese, Naava, Aviva and Nili. And this poem honors all the Bone Marrow Transplant doctors, nurses, techs, patients and their Donors!

And a special thank you to all the staff at the University of Maryland Marlene and Stewart Greenebaum Comprehensive Cancer Center for providing such amazing care!

# SUZIE Q GETS A BMT!

Once upon a time,
a long long time ago,
far far away,
in a land called C- A
there lived Loo
and a little girl named Suzie Q

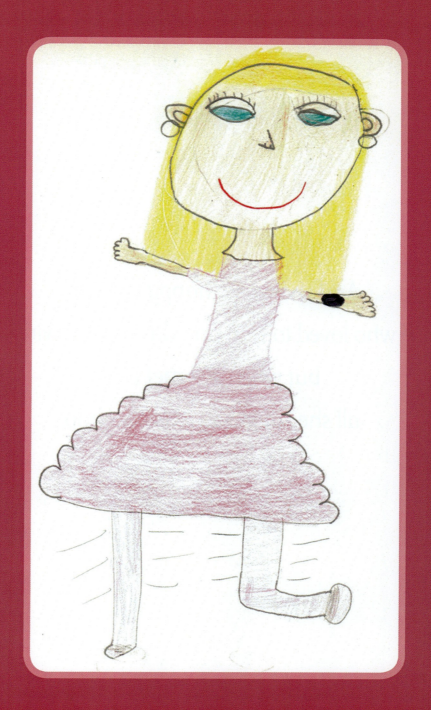

And she was a happy little girl,
who loved to sing and dance and twirl
but when she met Loo,
all she could say was boo-hoo.

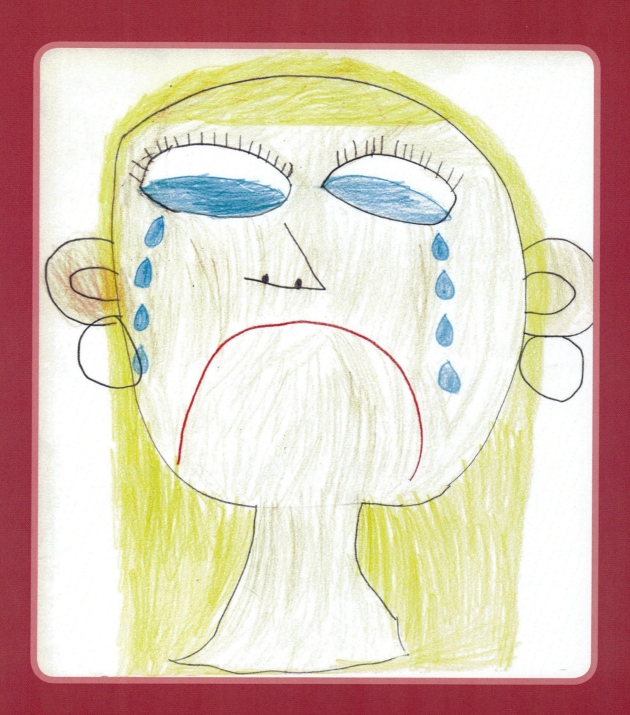

Loo was short for leukemia

acute lymphoblastic leukemia

in the land of C-A

Things felt different night and day,

A new doctor came to visit to say,

There would be a new treatment today.

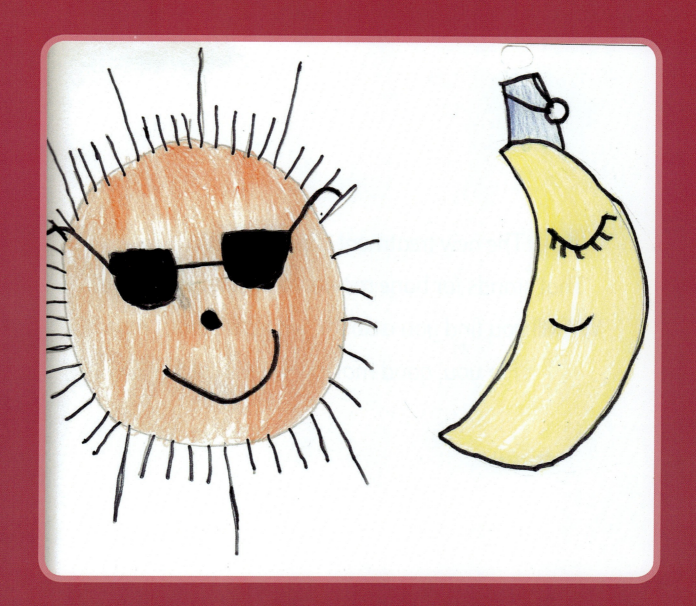

The new treatment is called a "BMT"

That stands for bone marrow transplant, you see

We will you find you a donor, who is a perfect match

For you, good marrow we will catch

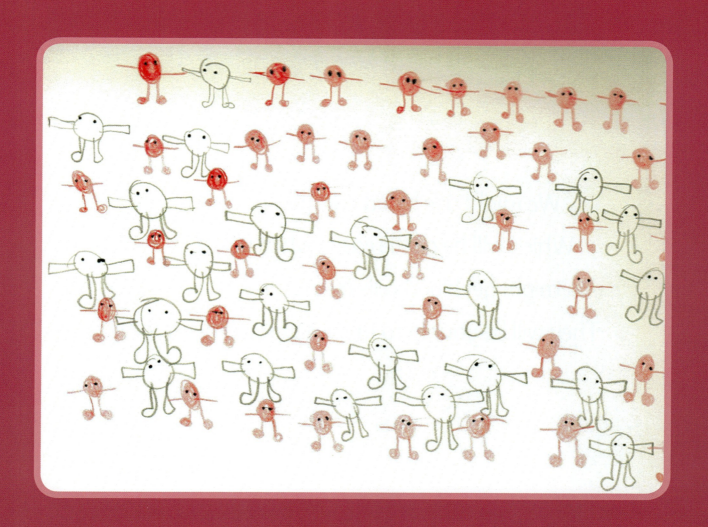

We might use blood cells that are your own

Which will be a little easier when you go home

Or, you might get blood cells from someone you never met,

They will be your hero forever, you will never forget.

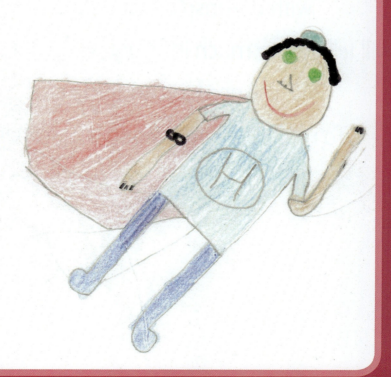

So you will have a new bunch of doctors,
with a transplant coordinator

They will tell you so much info, you will need a translator.

We will need to run some tests,

To make sure your body is at its best

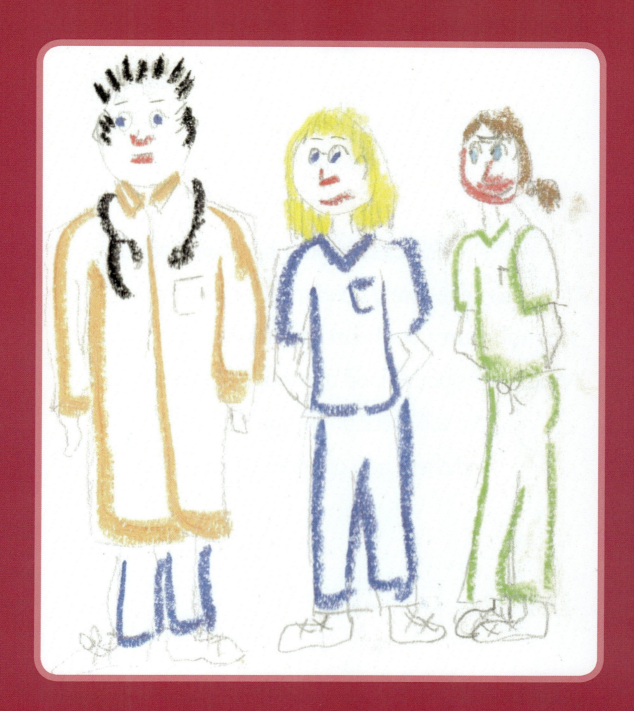

We will check how your heart will sound
To make sure a good match can be found.
To make sure your heart goes thump thump thump
And moves your blood around, pump pump pump
We will check your mouth and nose
And check you out down to your toes

thump

thump

thump

thump

15

We need to be sure all your body parts are good

And working the right way, like they should

You will *see* a dentist, pulmonologist, phlebotomist and a shrink

They will ask you questions and really make you think

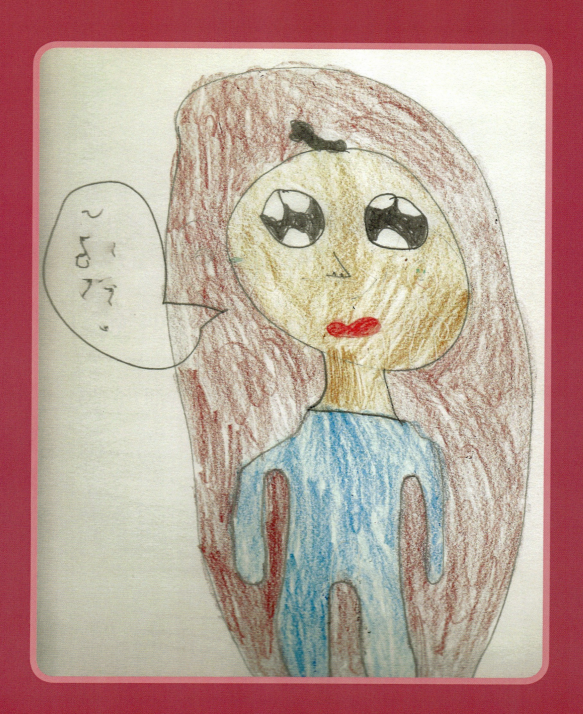

About all your dreams and goals, of
things to do when you grow up
And give you more chemo and you will throw-up!

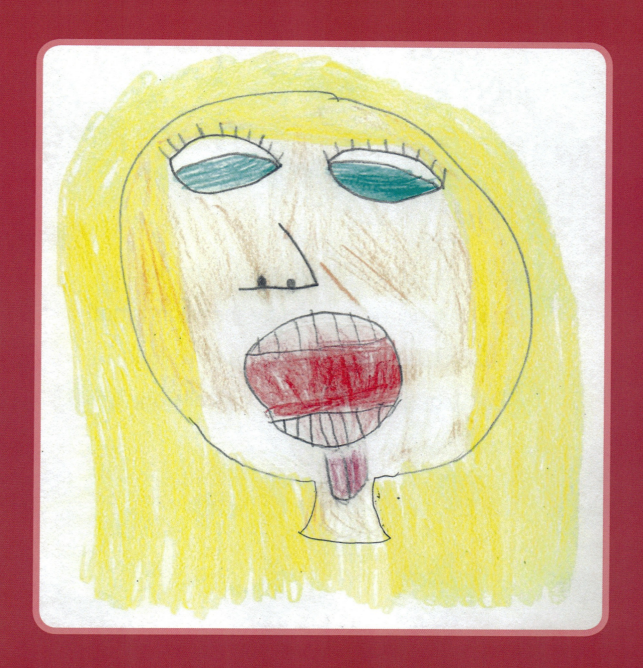

That's gross That's disgusting- Oh no not that!
Suzie Q lost her hair, and now she wears a hat!
Suzie Q used to have hair that was long
Pretty and blonde but now it's all gone.

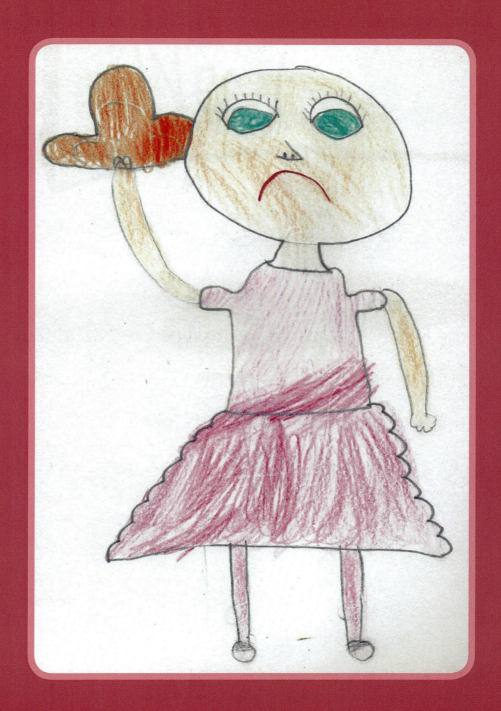

So the first thing we have to do

Is hold a blood drive for you

The Rabbi said we could do it in the shul lobby

Maybe there are folks who give blood for a hobby

Akiva set up his cameras for all to *see*

And folks even came out from the local TV.

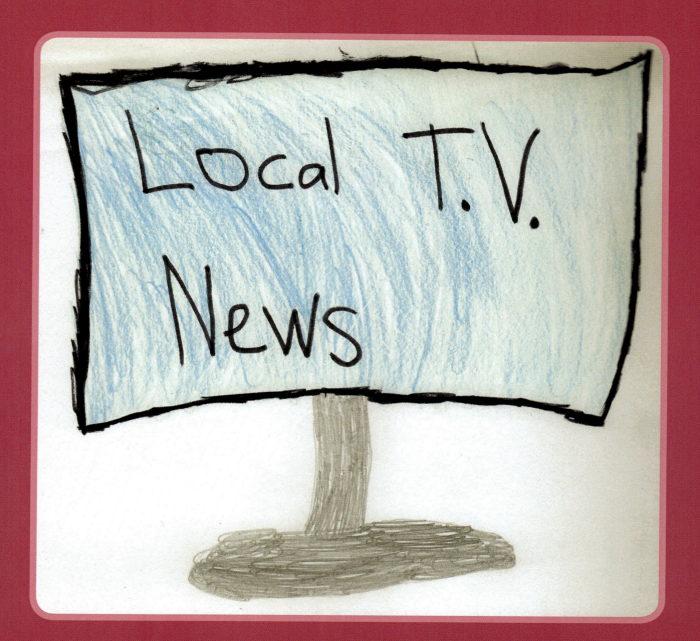

So then folks came from DKMS

Traveled to Baltimore from Texas

A nice lady named Amy,

Got all the materials for us

People drove from everywhere, some came by bus

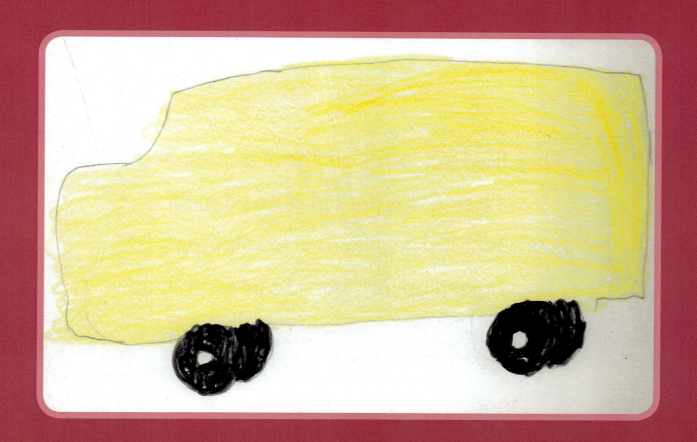

They filled out forms and gave a cheek swab

The shul was packed, it was a mob

Over 300 people came to volunteer

They offered up their bone marrow to share

But with cancer, that's just how it is
All these doctors, keep u really bizz
You might meet with a social worker, Like Dr. Sue
She says, "I'm Dr. Sue, I'm here for you!"

She will come visit and say "How are you?

"You can tell me anything you want to talk about

How this is scary, shocking, and you might want to shout!

I'm Dr. Sue, I'm here for you

Please tell me how you feel about all this,

About your family and friends, you will miss.

I'm Dr. Sue, I'm here for you

You won't get one needle from me,

or any medicine that tastes yucky."

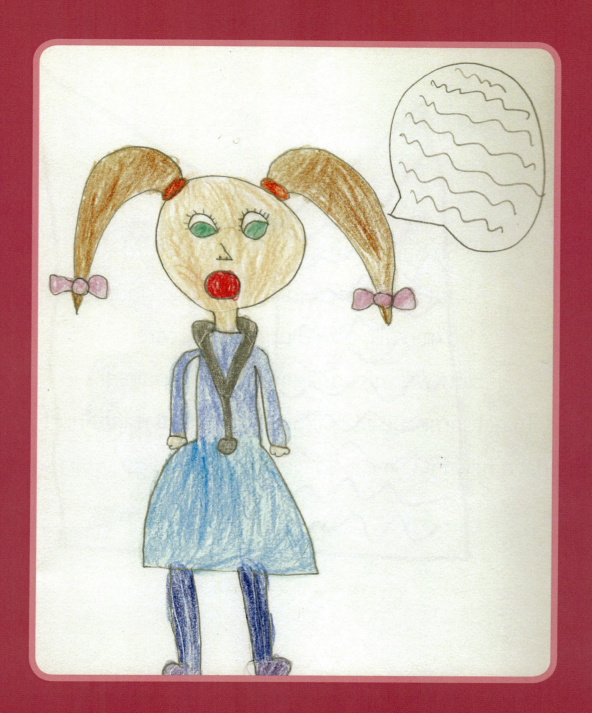

So Suzie Q thought long and hard

About her BMT, and let down her guard

"I'm really afraid and really scared,

How will my bone marrow be repaired?

To get someone else's blood in me, that might hurt

and get a new PICC line, and watch the blood go squirt squirt."

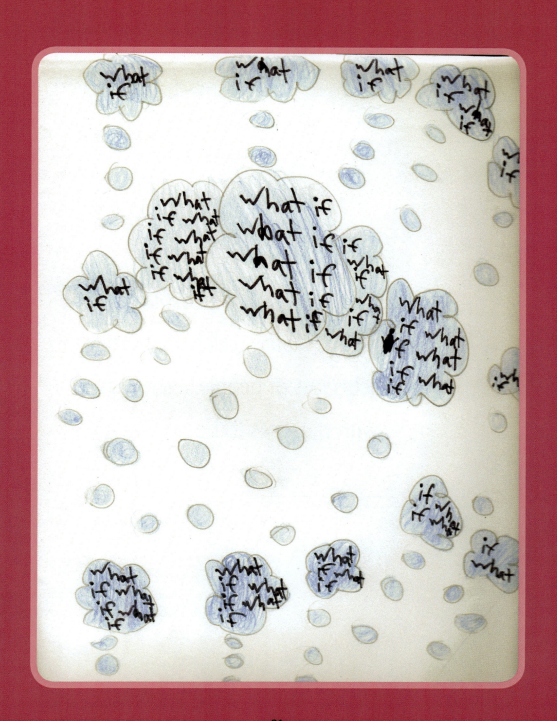

But a bone marrow transplant
is almost like a stem cell transplant
and it helps lots of people, even kids
with diseases to be rid

Hodgkin and non Hodgkins lymphoma
and multiple myeloma
ALL, CLL, AML, CML, lots of kinds of leukemia,
aplastic anemia and even sickle cell anemia
and immune deficiency disorders
or to keep solid tumors in their borders

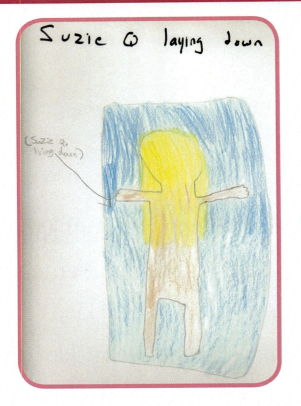

To prepare for the BMT, you have to focus,

on getting healthy, no playing hocus pocus

to make the bad cells disappear.

So soon good news we will hear.

There are a lot of things we have to do,

to get you ready to fix the bone marrow inside of you

Hocus Pocus Magic Tricks

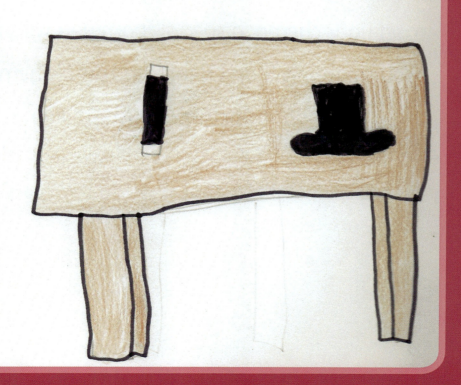

You might need to go to the infusion center
to get your chemo, a special room you will enter
You might need an LP for intrathecal chemo,
a lumbar puncture is the next step

Do Not
Enter

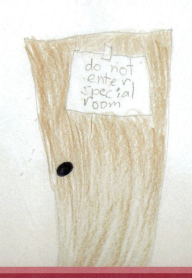

You have to stay still, you will have no pep

They will look in your spine up your back

And the bad cells they will attack

They will give you some meds, so you can sleep

so you don't make a sound, not even a peep

There is a worry that it may spread to your brain

The doctors will follow it, but not fly a plane

You might need to stay in the hospital bed

And will have time to get lots of book read

After the LP you will get more meds

You might feel like you are going crazy, like you have two heads

vincristine, cyterabine, methotrexate and steroids

voryconozole, proconozole, and the yellow paint

it is so much medicine

you might start to feel faint

Suzie Q with 2 Heads!

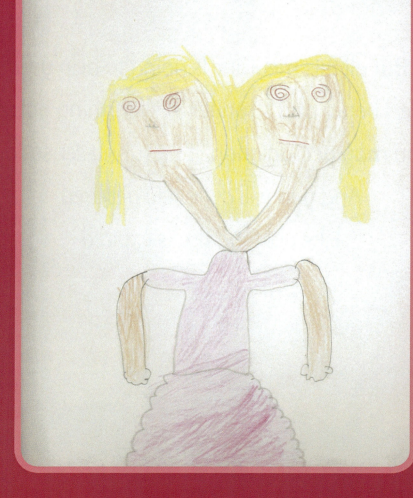

But all this medicine is going to help you

to feel better and stronger in everything you do

You may get radiation, it's a funny sensation

And you will definitely get tired

Like old food that's expired

Your pee may turn red or orange

UT-oh, nothing rhymes with orange.

So after induction and conditioning chemo,
the docs will say you are ready

to receive your BMT

Dr. Rapaport has to give the OK

he's here to save me today

All the nurses on the 9$^{th}$ floor really care,

they say don't come back Loo, Don't you dare

So nurses Sherri, Mindy, Tyler and Pat,

All stood up, they never sat

They watched the new cells go in the Picc line

Making sure we kept good time

A month later, it was time to leave

And ring the bell, I could finally breathe.

Jeff Adams, the social worker, runs the BMT group.

He keeps us all connected; he keeps us in the loop.

So now you are ready for the next part

To the Allo clinic you will start

That's when you get a new doc

who will be your rock

She is pretty and smart and nice

She knows you worked hard to pay the price

To prep for your BMT

To meet with Dr. Hardy

She says she will be on the 9$^{th}$ floor

And we can meet at the door

To check your labs and temp

So covid is not something you want to get!

At the front door, There's Duane with a big smile on his face

We can tell, we can to the right place!

Then Miss Kim takes my blood from the port,

it's like a new game, like playing a sport

Then come the nurses, Jessica, Kristina and Nadine

They are so patient and nice, not one is mean

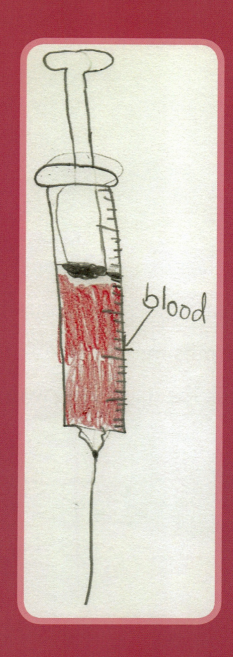

Next is the nurse practitioner, Susan

She is so wonderful, always movin',

She puts me on the table top,

And says "be still, so you won't drop"

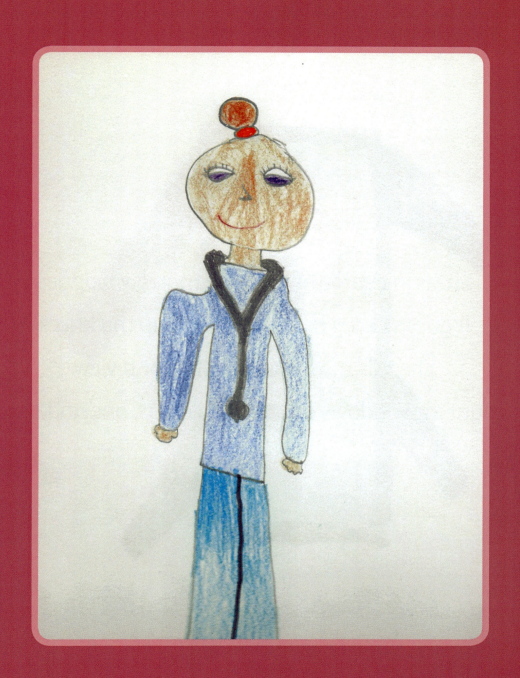

She is in charge of the bone marrow biopsies

It doesn't even hurt when I curl up my knees

She tells me to look outside for a view

count the windows on other buildings, one and two

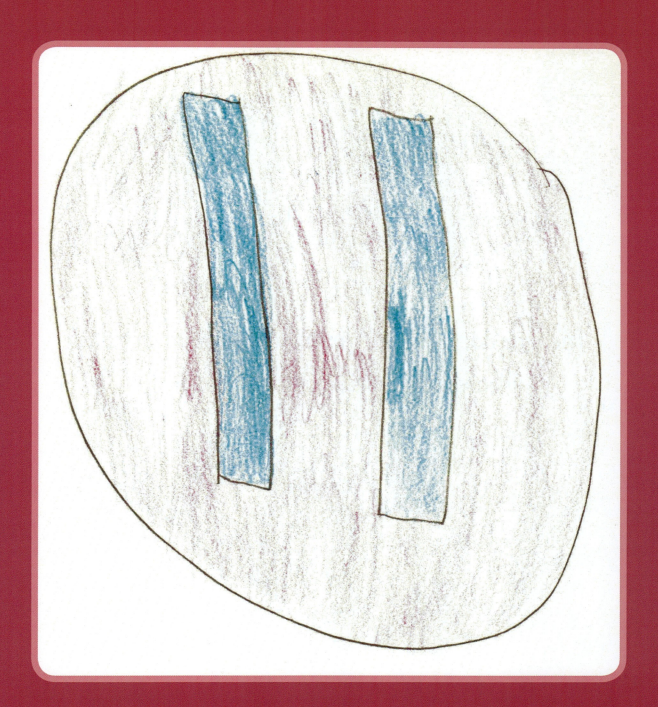

Then the doctor says, "I'm Dr Nancy Maureen Hardy. Please please please Come to my party!

We will *see* you three times a week
and after blood draws we can speak.

Suzie Q says, "Fancy Nancy, is that really you?

Will you help me get rid of Loo?

I have seen you in my library book

And this is exactly how you would look!'

Fancy Nancy - My new doctor

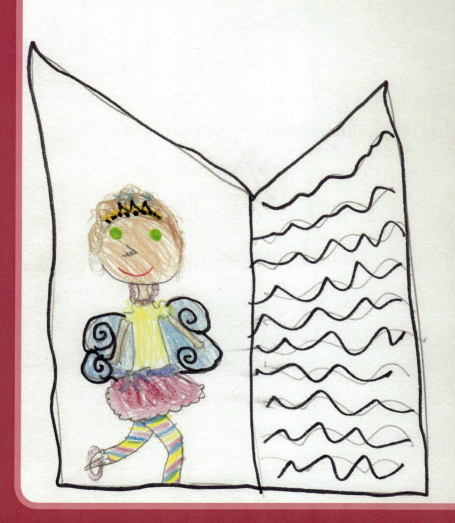

And now I have 100 per cent chimerism

The docs say I'm in remission

But I still have a suspicion

That Loo has not finished her mission

Loo says...

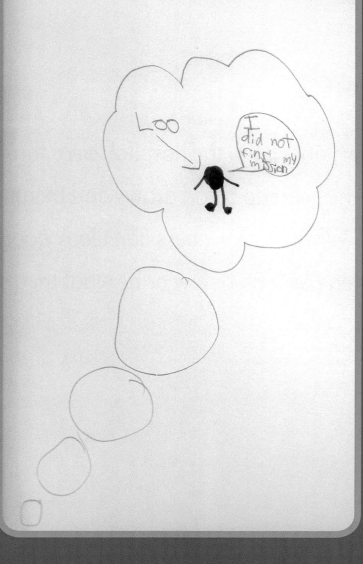

So now I only go to the hospital every fourth week

So they can do blood draws and then tweak

Whatever numbers don't look good

Or aren't as high or low or be what they should

Suzie Q starts to feel better

And she'd like to put all this in a shredder

To forget about all this pain

But then, Look at everything she has to gain

Suzie Q is much more spiritual

And less concerned with the material

She turns to G-d to pray,

and says to all "Have a nice day"

And means it in every way.

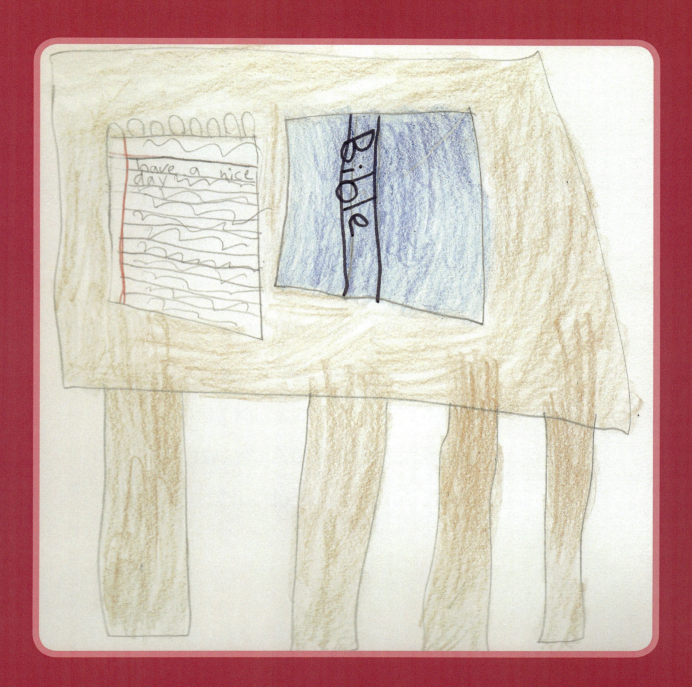

Stay healthy, Be positive. Life is so special

Eat fruits and veggies, maybe a pretzel

Change your attitude

Always show gratitude

Say please and thank you

for everything others do for you.

Always remember to Apologize

if you feel a funny noise about to arise

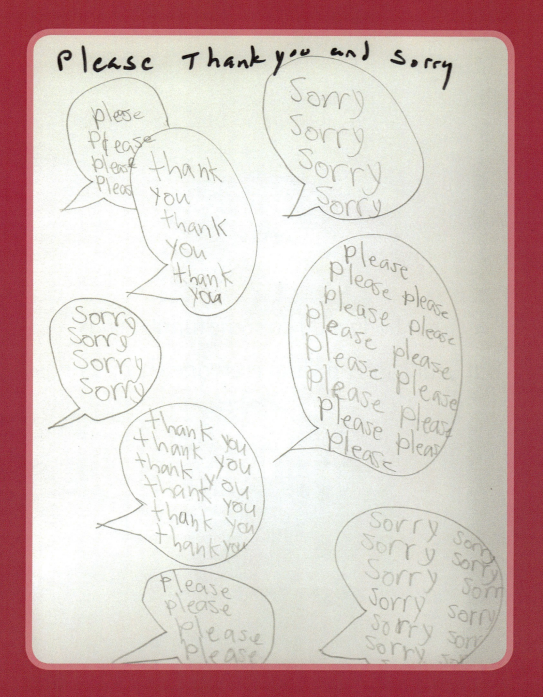

Your body may do some funny things

But your cancer pulls at everyone's heartstrings.

So go enjoy your new BMT
you have new blood in your body
Soon you will be as good as new
And let the doctors follow you

Suzie Q has met so many nice folks

She apologizes for the fun she pokes

Maybe one day, in the future, you too

Will write about a book, about all you have been through!

# Writing my journal

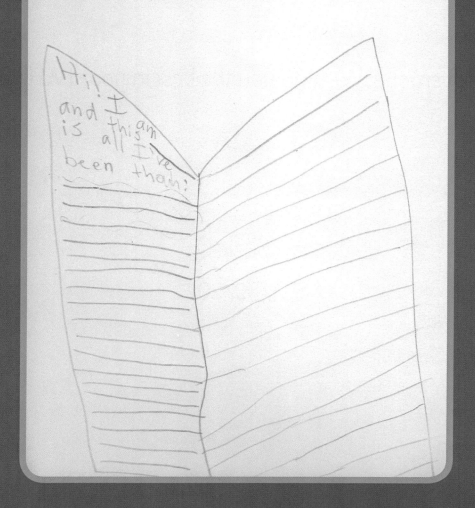

Hi! I am
and this
is all I've
been than!

Be well everyone. Wishing you the best in your BMT recovery.


Suzie Q

11/30/2021

Printed in the United States
by Baker & Taylor Publisher Services